# What If?
# by Randall Munroe

: This is a quick read summary based on the novel
"What If"
by Randall Munroe

# NOTE TO READERS:

This is a Summary & Analysis of What If by Randall Munroe. You are encouraged to buy the full version.

**Copyright** 2016 **by** ABookADay. All rights reserved worldwide. No part of this publication may be reproduced or transmitted in any form without the prior written consent of the publisher.

# TABLE OF CONTENTS

ANALYSIS

OVERVIER

SUMMARY

Question 1: What would happen if the Earth and all terrestrial objects suddenly stopped spinning, but the atmosphere retained its velocity?

Question 2: What would happen if you tried to hit a baseball pitched at 90 percent the speed of light?

Question 3: What if I took a swim in a typical spent nuclear fuel pool? Would I need to dive to actually experience a fatal amount of radiation? How long could I stay safely at the surface?

Question 4: I assume when you travel back in time you end up at the same spot on the Earth's surface. At least, that's how it worked in the *Back to the Future* movies. If so, what would it be like if you traveled back in time, starting in Times Square, New York, 1000 years? 10,000 years? 100,000 years? 1,000,000 years? 1,000,000,000 years? What about forward in time 1,000,000 years?

Question 5: What if everyone actually had only one soul mate, a random person somewhere in the world?

Question 6: If every person on Earth aimed a laser pointer at the Moon at the same time, would it change color?

Question 7: What would happen if you made a periodic table out of cube-shaped bricks, where each brick was made of the corresponding element?

Question 8: What would happen if everyone on Earth stood as close to each other as they could and jumped, everyone landing on the ground at the same instant?

Question 9: What would happen if you were able to gather a mole (unit of measurement) of moles (the small furry critter) in one place?

Question 10: What would happen if a hair dryer with continuous power were turned on and put in an airtight 1 x 1 x 1-meter box?

Question 11: If every human somehow simply disappeared from the face of the Earth, how long would it be before the last artificial light source would go out?

Question 12: Is it possible to build a jetpack using downward-firing machine guns?

Question 13: If you suddenly began rising steadily at 1 foot per second, how exactly would you die? Would you freeze or suffocate first? Or something else?

Question 14: How long could a nuclear submarine last in orbit?

Questions 15-21: Short Answer

Question 22: Lightning

Question 23: How much computing power could we achieve if the entire world population stopped whatever we are doing right now and started doing calculations? How would it compare to a modern-day computer or smartphone?

Question 24: If an asteroid was very small but supermassive, could you really live on it like the Little Prince?

Question 25: From what height would you need to drop a steak for it to be cooked when it hit the ground?

Question 26: How hard would a puck have to be shot to be able to knock the goalie himself backward into the net?

Question 27: If everyone on the planet stayed away from each other for a couple of weeks, wouldn't the common cold be wiped out?

Question 28: What if a glass of water was, all of a sudden, literally half empty?

Question 29: Let's assume there's life on the nearest habitable exoplanet and that they have technology comparable to ours. If they looked at our star right now, what would they see?

Question 30: This may be a bit gruesome, but...if someone's DNA suddenly vanished, how long would that person last?

Question 31: What would happen if you tried to fly a normal Earth airplane above different solar system bodies?

Question 32: How much Force power can Yoda output?

Question 33: Which U.S. state is actually flown over the most?

Question 34: What if I jumped out of an airplane with a couple of tanks of helium and one huge, un-inflated balloon? Then, while falling, I release the helium and fill the balloon. How long of a fall would I need in order for the balloon to slow me enough that I could land safely?

Question 35: Is there enough energy to move the entire current human population off-planet?

Question 36: I read about some researchers who were trying to produce sperm from bone marrow stem cells. If a woman were to have sperm cells made from her own stem cells and impregnate herself, what would be her relationship to her daughter?

Question 37: How high can a human throw something?

Question 38: How close would you have to be to a supernova to get a lethal dose of neutrino radiation?

Question 39: How fast can you hit a speed bump while driving and live?

Question 40: If two immortal people were placed on opposite sides of an uninhabited Earthlike planet, how long would it take them to find each other? 100,000 years? 1,000,000 years? 100,000,000,000 years?

Questions 41-43: Orbital speed

Question 44: When—if ever—will the bandwidth of the Internet surpass that of FedEx?

Question 45: What place on Earth would allow you to free-fall the longest by jumping off it? What about using a squirrel suit?

Question 46: In the movie *300* they shoot arrows up into the sky and they seemingly blot out the sun. Is this possible, and how many arrows would it take?

Question 47: How quickly would the oceans drain if a circular portal 10 meters in radius leading into space were created at the bottom of Challenger Deep, the deepest spot in the ocean? How would the Earth change as the water was being drained?

Question 48: Supposing you did drain the oceans, and dumped the water on top of the *Curiosity* rover, how would Mars change as the water accumulated?

Question 49: How many unique English tweets are possible? How long would it take for the population of the world to read them all out loud?

Question 50: How many Lego bricks would it take to build a bridge capable of carrying traffic from London to New York? Have that many Lego bricks been manufactured?

Question 51: What is the longest possible sunset you can experience while driving, assuming we are obeying the speed limit and driving on paved roads?

Question 52: If you call a random phone number and say "God bless you," what are the chances that the person who answers just sneezed?

Question 53: How long would it take for people to notice their weight gain if the mean radius of the world expanded by 1cm every second?

Question 54: Assuming a zero-gravity environment with an atmosphere identical to Earth's, how long would it take the friction of air to stop an arrow fired from a bow? Would it eventually come to a standstill and hover in midair?

Question 55: What would happen to the Earth if the Sun suddenly switched off?

Question 56: If you had a printed version of the whole of (say, the English) Wikipedia, how many printers would you need in order to keep up with the changes made to the live version?

Question 57: When, if ever, will Facebook contain more profiles of dead people than living ones?

Question 58: When (if ever) did the Sun finally set on the British Empire?

Question 59: I was absentmindedly stirring a cup of hot tea, when I got to thinking, "Aren't I actually adding kinetic energy into this cup?" I know that stirring does help to cool down the tea, but what if I were to stir it faster? Would I be able to boil a cup of water by stirring?

Question 60: If all the lightning strikes happening in the world on any given day all happened in the same place at once, what would happen to that place?

Question 61: What is the farthest one human being has ever been from every other living person? Were they lonely?

Question 62: What if a rainstorm dropped all of its water in a single giant drop?

Question 63: What if everyone who took the SAT guessed on every multiple choice question? How many perfect scores would there be?

Question 64: If a bullet with the density of a neutron star were fired from a handgun (ignoring the how) at the Earth's surface, would the Earth be destroyed?

Question 65: What if a Richter magnitude 15 earthquake were to hit America at, let's say, New York City? What about a Richter 20? 25?

ANALYSIS

# ANALYSIS

*The questions in these sections are some of the strangest the author has received. In response, the author provides a humorous cartoon to both answer and acknowledge the absurdity of these questions. These questions are not covered in the following summary as the responses are purely visual.

# OVERVIEW

This review of *What If: Serious Scientific Answers to Absurd Hypothetical Questions* by Randall Munroe provides a chapter by chapter detailed summary followed by an analysis and critique of the strengths and weaknesses of the book.

The main theme explored in the book is how we can use science as a way to answer some of life's strangest and most unanswerable questions. Using data gathered from various sources such as clinical studies, scientific journal articles, and interviews with top scientific and analytical minds, the author is able to a provide answers to his audience's most absurd questions.

The central thesis of the work is that any question humans have ever had about the way the world works or possible ramifications if the world stopped working the way we expect it to can all be answered through scientific means. Munroe takes each question from his audience and thoroughly examines it—mostly reserving judgement—and attempts to find the best answer possible. In some cases, he provides several different answers, and in others even provides answers to questions that the audience did not ask, but are related to the subject at hand. What makes his responses unique is that he relies on humor (and cartoons) to explain even the most difficult concepts and this allows for his answers to be easily understood by all of his audience, even those with no scientific background.

Randall Munroe is the writer and creator of the web comic xkcd and has written a previous book of the same title. He worked at NASA as a roboticist until October of 2006 when he became a professional web comic artist full time. *What If?* is the result of his popular web comic and a project inspired by it where he asked users to post absurd math and physics related questions. He currently resides in Cambridge, Massachusetts.

# SUMMARY

**Introduction**

## QUESTION 1: WHAT WOULD HAPPEN IF THE EARTH AND ALL TERRESTRIAL OBJECTS SUDDENLY STOPPED SPINNING, BUT THE ATMOSPHERE RETAINED ITS VELOCITY?

First, the author explains, everyone would die. Then, because the Earth moves on its axis at over a thousand miles per hour, if it stopped and the air did not, this would create a thousand-mile-per-hour wind. These supersonic winds would only last a few seconds, but wipe out all human structures. The author suggests that not every human would be killed by these winds, but rather by the debris. He suggests that the only hope of surviving this would be to be in Helsinki, Finland (or at the

Amundsen-Scott research station at the South Pole). This is because these locations are at a high enough latitude away from the equator that the winds would not be as harsh. In Helsinki in particular, the bedrock below has a complex system of tunnels where one could completely survive underground.

Once the winds die down, the air around it will heat up and creating scorching temperatures and global thunderstorms. While this is occurring, the author postulates, the wind that has swept over the ocean will have picked up most of the coldest ocean water and mix with the superheated air. Not only will this kill any life form in the ocean (really, any life form that needs to breathe), but it will send huge tsunamis across the shores of all continents.

Because the Earth has stopped, we will lose our usual night/day cycles. As the Sun would still be moving, we would experience a full rising and setting over the course of one year. So, one half of the Earth will experience daytime, scorching constant sunlight, for six months. Then, for the remaining six months, it would experience plummeting temperatures, exasperated by the dense blanket of fog created by the sheer amount of dust and debris kicked up into the atmosphere from the windstorm. The author likens the atmosphere to that of an early Venus.

Also, our Moon, lacking our rotation to feed it's tidal energy, will begin coming towards us. As it grows closer, it's tides would begin to accelerate our spin and it's gravity will slowly force us to start turning once more. The Earth's rotation would start anew, but humans would no longer be alive to experience it.

# QUESTION 2: WHAT WOULD HAPPEN IF YOU TRIED TO HIT A BASEBALL PITCHED AT 90 PERCENT THE SPEED OF LIGHT?

The author imagines that the ball would move so fast that even the molecules around it would become still. The ball would hit the air molecules so hard that they would fuse with the atoms of the ball's surface and create a bubble of plasma. This fusion would naturally slow the ball down, but because it is already going so fast, it would eat away at the ball and send tiny fragments of it in all directions. These fragments would hit the air so hard that they would create several blasts of fusion. Essentially, once this ball reaches the batter (which he would never even see), it is a bullet-shaped cloud of plasma, hitting him first with x-rays, then the cloud of debris. It would literally disintegrate the batter, audience, and stadium in the first microsecond. There would be an immense fireball, mushroom cloud, and blast wave taking down everything within a mile of the park.

# Question 3: What if I took a swim in a typical spent nuclear fuel pool? Would I need to dive to actually experience a fatal amount of radiation? How long could I stay safely at the surface?

First, Munroe imagines, you might be able to tread water for roughly 10-40 hours before you blackout and drown. Despite that, he explains that you would be pretty safe because water is very good at shielding radiation, this is why were keep nuclear reactor fuel at the bottom of pools until it is inert. He gives a visual diagram of how one of these pools looks and explains that every seven centimeters of water cuts radiation in half, showing a "region of danger" as you get closer to the fuel rods.

Oddly, treading water in one of these pools will likely give you less radiation exposure than if you walked near it, simply because of how water absorbs the dose. The only issue would be if there was corrosion in one of the fuel rods, but even then it is safe enough to swim in (yet, not enough to drink).

To further prove the shielding effects of water, Munroe cites an example from August 31, 2010, when a diver was servicing a spent fuel pool in Switzerland. He found a length of tubing at the bottom of the pool and was instructed to take it up in his tool basket. As he lifted it out of the water, the radiation alarms went off, and he dropped it back in and got out. His body, particularly his right hand, showed that it had been exposed to a higher than normal amount of radiation. It turns out this tube had fallen off of a rod four years prior and was so radioactive that if he had placed it close to his body, he would have been killed. The water literally protected him from the radiation.

# Question 4: I assume when you travel back in time you end up at the same spot on the Earth's surface. At least, that's how it worked in the *Back to the Future* movies. If so, what would it be like if you traveled back in time, starting in Times Square, New York, 1000 years? 10,000 years? 100,000 years? 1,000,000 years? 1,000,000,000 years? What about forward in time 1,000,000 years?

Going 1000 years back, the author suggests that we look at a project called Welikia, which has produced a detailed ecological map of New York City during the time of the arrival of the Europeans. Times Square would likely look like an old-growth forest, there would be more large animals (including wolves and mountain lions), more chestnut trees (as there was a blight during the early twentieth century), and—oddly—no earthworms.

Going 10,000 years back, Earth was coming out of a great cold period as great ice sheets were withdrawing all the way back across the Canadian border, scouring the land down to its bedrock. Life began moving back north (with the exception of the earthworms). Large chunks of ice broke off of the ice sheets and melted, creating kettlehole ponds like what we see as today's Oakland Lake in Queens. Boulders, called glacial erratics, would be left behind by the ice sheets, and as the ice melted, rivers of water flowed under the sheets, carrying gravel and sand and often creating large ridges called eskers.

Going 100,000 years back, Earth was at the end of it's Sangamon interglacial period which supported a stable climate and an ecology probably very similar to our own. Coastal geography and the locations of some islands would be different, and there would be a variety of unusual kinds of animals. This includes the pronghorn, the dire wolf, the short-faced bear, and the saber-toothed cat.

Going 1,000,000 years back, the world is in its Quaternary period and the climate is relatively stable and warm. Our new animals were joined by a long-limbed hyena, which does not just reside in Africa, but also North America.

Going 1,000,000,000 years back, the continental plates are pushed together into a supercontinent called Rodinia where Manhattan was probably connected to Angola and South Africa. There are no plants or animals here, and there is only single-cell life in the oceans. The surface of the water is covered in cyanobacteria which breathe in carbon dioxide and breathe out oxygen that is toxic to all other life forms, causing an oxygen catastrophe. Creatures evolve from this that can breath in oxygen, and this is where we evolve from.

Going 1,000,000 years forward, it is likely that humans will have died out. Earth's geology will continue on and eventually glaciers will advance once more. While all human artifacts will have faded, it is likely that only the layer of plastic we've deposited over the planet will remain.

In the far future, as the Sun is gradually brightening, our oceans will boil away and surround the planet in a thick water vapor, creating another Venus. Our crust will eventually also boil and we will ultimately be consumed by the Sun. The author suggests that if we do manage to escape the Earth and find life outside of the solar system, our descendants may one day live on a planet built from the dust clouds of our incinerated Earth.

# Question 5: What if everyone actually had only one soul mate, a random person somewhere in the world?

Assuming your soul mate is chosen at birth, it is unlikely that they will even still be alive as a hundred billion or so humans have already lived and only seven billion live now. You would also have to increase the possibly that they could be a human that will exist in the future. However, even if your soul mate lived now, and was within a few years of age as yourself, there would still be a pool of around half a billion potential mates.

The author adds in questions of gender, sexual orientation, culture, language, etc. to narrow it down, but ultimately pushes against these restrictions as the questions suggests a completely random soul mate. With this, the odds of running in to them are very small as even if you lock eyes with a few dozen strangers a day (and with only 10% being around your age) that is still only seeing 50,000 people in a lifetime: and there are 500,000,000 potential soul mates in the world.

The author suggests a conveyer belt of sorts, even a webcam, where you could make eye contact for a few seconds with a person to determine if they are your soul mate. Using this eight hours a day, seven days a week, you could be matched up with your soul mate in just a few decades. It is likely that people would feel so much pressure to find their soul mate, that they would feel the need to fake it with someone they did not care about. Ultimately, it would be a very lonely world.

# Question 6: If every person on Earth aimed a laser pointer at the Moon at the same time, would it change color?

Because not everyone can see the Moon at once, we would first need to choose on spot where the Moon is visible to as many people as possible: ideally when the moon is over the Arabian Sea. Also, we would need to choose a quarter moon so we can see the effect of the lasers on both the light and dark sides. With a typical five milliwatt laser, there would be no effect because Sunlight will far outshine the lasers. Using a one watt laser (capable of burning human skin), there will still be no effect. Using a NightSun (a searchlight used by the police and Coast Guard) which gives off 50,000 lumens, there is a barely discernable difference. Increasing the power by using a 30,000 watt IMAX projector array there is still a barely noticeable difference. It is not until you increase the power to the most powerful spotlight on Earth—the Luxor Beam—that you have a visible light on the moon.

Adding more power by shining a megawatt chemical oxygen iodine laser (used by the Department of Defense to destroy incoming missiles) we are finally able to match the power of the Sun, but it would use up half the Earth's supply of electricity and burn up in about two minutes. If we implausibly were able to use an ultraviolet laser, like the confinement beam at the National Ignition Facility, it would put out 500 terawatts and, in all scenarios, would light the Earth on fire. Ultimately, firing this laser at the Moon would send it rocketing into space, hitting the Sun, the other planets, and be swung around it's orbit, slamming it into Earth.

## QUESTION 7: WHAT WOULD HAPPEN IF YOU MADE A PERIODIC TABLE OUT OF CUBE-SHAPED BRICKS, WHERE EACH BRICK WAS MADE OF THE CORRESPONDING ELEMENT?

Out of the 118 elements, it is only possible to get samples of 80 (90 if you are willing to risk your own safety and health) as the rest are extremely radioactive. Ignoring this, you could stack the first two rows without much trouble. In row one, only Hydrogen and Helium would rise and disperse. In row two you would have issues with Fluorine as it is the most corrosive and reactive element in the table and you would most certainly need a gas mask to avoid breathing in trace amounts.

The third row will certainly burn you because of the Phosphorus, which, when next to Sulfur, Fluorine and Chlorine, it will catch fire. This will create other chemicals that will choke you with toxic smoke. Row four will also kill you with toxic smoke as the burning Phosphorus will ignite the Arsenic. Row five, with it's Technetium-99, will help in doing all of these things while also giving you a hefty dose of radiation.

Row six contains many radioactive elements like Promethium, Polonium, Astatine, and Radon. Ultimately, even the mere presence of Astatine would cause an explosion of radiation. Lastly, the seventh row has transuranic elements that are so unstable that they can only exist for a few minutes at a time. In doing so, they will decay radioactively and release so much energy that there would be a nuclear explosion.

Munroe's answer is, quite simply, do not do this.

## QUESTION 8: WHAT WOULD HAPPEN IF EVERYONE ON EARTH STOOD AS CLOSE TO EACH OTHER AS THEY COULD AND JUMPED, EVERYONE LANDING ON THE GROUND AT THE SAME INSTANT?

For this, all the people would essentially need to be standing on Rhode Island. After crunching the numbers and full examining the scenario, Munroe admits that ultimately nothing would happen as the Earth greatly outweighs us. Even the energy delivered into the Earth is spread out over such an area that it really does not do much.

In examining this, however, the author suggests a deeper look into this scenario, realizing the consequences of having every person on Earth in Rhode Island, and having nothing happen when they attempt this experiment. He suggest that after the experiment, everyone would attempt to use their cell phones to see if anything happened across the Earth—effectively collapsing the cell networks, and then causing a global traffic jam as everyone tries to leave Rhode Island at the same time. This would cause chaos and violence leading into an apocalyptic scenario where the human species is decimated and the Earth itself is left completely empty, yet ultimately physically unaltered.

# Question 9: What would happen if you were able to gather a mole (unit of measurement) of moles (the small furry critter) in one place?

The unit of measurement of the mole is 602,214,129,000,000,000,000,000, which means there would be this many burrowing mammals in one space. This many moles would weigh nearly as much as a planet, so doing this on Earth is not possible. The author suggests doing this in interplanetary space, where gravity would pull them into a sphere. Essentially, the moles would die and decompose, giving off heat. It would break down into a mush or organic matter that could eventually form oil. These moles would disgustingly turn into a giant planet of dead mole meat. Due to their fur coats, the moles would trap the heat inward, periodically releasing blasts of air up to the surface, causing some mole bodies to be freed from the planet. After centuries of this, the planet would cool off enough to freeze through and be a solid dead-meat planet.

# Question 10: What would happen if a hair dryer with continuous power were turned on and put in an airtight 1 x 1 x 1-meter box?

First, the author clarifies that a hair dryer draws in 1874 watts of power. This means that it will also give off the same amount. The inside of the box it is placed in will grow hotter and hotter, until the outer surface will soon begin to give off heat. Normally, this would burn out the hair dryer. But, if it is indestructible, the author gleefully tests just how hot he can make the hair dryer, examining each of the effects the hotter it goes. Going all the way up to 1.875 gigawatts, the author draws on *Back to the Future* and suggests that the hair dryer is drawing in so much energy that it could travel back in time. Even taking it up to 11 petwatts (far beyond the amount of power consumed by every other electrical device on the planet combined), the author suggests that the box would heat up so much that it would rise into the air, shoot through the atmosphere and leave most of the Earth burning in it's wake.

# Question 11: If every human somehow simply disappeared from the face of the Earth, how long would it be before the last artificial light source would go out?

A majority of the lights would go down when the power grids do—which would be very quickly as the fossil fuel plants that provide most of the world's electricity require humans to run them. The author then goes in to detail about what would happen to several different energy sources we use for light on Earth.

Diesel generators, which service remote areas such as islands, would operate until they ran out of fuel (anywhere between a few days to a couple of months). Geothermal plants are powered by the Earth's internal heat and could run for a few years until they would eventually corrode from disrepair. Wind turbines can run up to three years without maintenance and could possibly even continue for decades until they too would break down. Hydroelectric dams could also run for several years until they were eventually clogged or shut down by mechanical failure. Battery powered devices would also shut down in a few decades as, even in disuse, they self-discharge. Nuclear reactors could hypothetically continue running indefinitely if they were on a low-power mode, but it is likely that something would go wrong and the core will automatically shut down as a safety precaution. Space probes could last the longest but would be shut down in a few centuries due to conditions on other planets, space debris, satellite orbits decaying, or the voltage on the rovers dropping too low. Solar power, on the other hand, could easily last a century, so long as it is kept free from dust and corrosion by occasional winds and rain.

While this would technically be the last source for artificial light, there is still Cherenkov radiation which is the blue glow of nuclear reactor cores. This glow could easily last more than 200 years.

# Question 12: Is it possible to build a jetpack using downward-firing machine guns?

Yes. An AK-47 has a thrust-to-weight ratio of two, meaning that the recoil is larger than the weight of the gun (not true of all machine guns). The force of the gun pushing out a bullet, gas, and explosive debris, can accelerate it up to 30 percent higher. With this, the author explains that the AK-47 could take off, but would not be able to lift anything heavier than a squirrel and it's flight would only last about three seconds. By using at least 300 AK-47s at once, with 250 rounds of ammunition each, you could make it about a half a kilometer into the air.

Then, the author (always wanting to push more) investigates using bigger machine guns, ultimately arriving at the Russian made Gryazev-Shipunov GSh-6-30. It has a thrust-to-weight ratio of 40 and, insuring that everything is double guarded for safety, it could potentially be used to jump over mountains.

## Question 13: If you suddenly began rising steadily at 1 foot per second, how exactly would you die? Would you freeze or suffocate first? Or something else?

A foot per second is actually slower than an elevator, so it would take a long time to reach a dangerous height. It is not until about two hours in (when you are at about two kilometers up in the air) would you begin to reach below freezing temperatures and air pressures even lower than in an airplane cabin. As you continue up, the temperature would be your biggest issue and you would be most likely to die from hypothermia before oxygen deprivation. At 8000 meters up the oxygen content in the air would be too low for human life (earning it the nickname the Death Zone) and this would occur near the seven hour mark, where there would be no chance at all for survival.

# Question 14: How long could a nuclear submarine last in orbit?

The submarine itself would be fine as it is meant to withstand severe external pressure from water. The crew inside would be in danger of lack of oxygen, as there would be no water to extract oxygen from and they would need to use up all their reserves of it in just a few days. The submarine could also not maintain it's internal temperature due to lack of the ocean environment, so they would run out of warmth very quickly.

# Questions 15-21: Short Answer

**If my printer could literally print out money, would it have that big an effect on the world?**

The author explains that you could theoretically print $200 million dollars a year, but that is barely a dent in the world economy as there are nearly a billion hundred dollar bills printed each year.

**What would happen if you set off a nuclear bomb in the eye of a hurricane? Would the storm cell be immediately vaporized?**

Munroe cites the National Oceanic and Atmospheric Administration's response to this question: "Needless to say, this is not a good idea."

**If everyone put little turbine generators on the downspouts of their houses and businesses, how much power would we generate? Would we ever**

**generate enough power to offset the cost of the generators?**

Even in the rainiest part of the country, during the rainiest hour on record, the power gained would still not save a hundred dollars in less than a hundred years.

**Using only pronounceable letter combinations, how long would names have to be to give each star in the universe a unique one-word name?**

By alternating vowels and consonants, then each pair of letters added allows you to name 105 more stars. With about three sextillion stars in the universe, the names would be about as long as the same number of stars.

**I bike to class sometimes. It's annoying biking in the wintertime, because it's so cold. How fast would I have to bike for my skin to warm up the way a spacecraft heats up during reentry?**

You would need to increase the temperature of the air layer in front of your body by 20 degrees Celsius (from freezing to room temperature), and you can do this by going as fast as 200 meters per second.

## How much physical space does the Internet take up?

The author calculates this by how much the storage space industry produces, which is 650 million hard drives a year. He estimates it at eight liters, or two gallons, per second. In the past year's usage, this would amount to filling an oil tanker.

## What if you strapped C4 to a boomerang? Could this be an effective weapon, or would it be as stupid as it sounds?

The author responds with his own question: how could it be advantageous to have this kind of weapon come back at you if it misses it's target?

# Question 22: Lightning

**How dangerous is it, really, to be in a pool during a thunderstorm?**

This is mostly dangerous because of how conductive water is, and also the fact that a pool is a flat surface, where the amps of a bolt of lightning can easily spread outward. Even standing in a puddle of water would be dangerous.

**What would happen if you were in a boat or plane that got hit by lightning? Or a submarine?**

A boat with a cabin would be as safe as a car, while one without a cabin would be like being on a golf course. A submarine would be very safe.

**What would happen if lightning struck a bullet in midair?**

The bullet would not affect the lightning, and because the bolt and the bullet would be moving so fast, not much would happen to the bullet itself besides heating up a few degrees.

# Question 23: How much computing power could we achieve if the entire world population stopped whatever we are doing right now and started doing calculations? How would it compare to a modern-day computer or smartphone?

Munroe explains that this is a complicated question because humans and computers think differently, and human have specifically evolved to understand and expect certain outcomes and behaviors that computers have to be told to expect. However, using the same benchmarks that we test computers on, human beings have been surpassed by computers since as long ago as 1994, when Intel created their new Pentium chips.

Looking at computing benchmarks another way, he explains that the combined power of all computers against all the computing power of humans possibly surpassed us as long ago as 1977. Another examination could claim that computers could not be as complex as us until the year 2036. Ultimately, none of these answers matter as by 2014 we managed to reach the same combined complexity as that of the world's population of ants brains.

# Question 24: If an asteroid was very small but supermassive, could you really live on it like the Little Prince?

In order for this to be possible, an asteroid with a radius of about 1.75 meters would need to have a mass of about 500 million tons (the combined mass of every human being). Because of this, anyone living on the planet would need to avoid running too fast, as they may be sent into orbit.

# Question 25: From what height would you need to drop a steak for it to be cooked when it hit the ground?

The author examines how a steak might be cooked when dropped from increasingly higher altitudes, finding that it would do things such as char, freeze, and shatter. Ultimately, even if the steak were dropped from the edge of our atmosphere, it would slowly disintegrate as it's outer layer is repeatedly charred and broken off by wind blasts but still remain raw on the inside.

# Question 26: How hard would a puck have to be shot to be able to knock the goalie himself backward into the net?

This can not happen as human hockey players are much heavier than hockey pucks. Several factors make this impossible: a hockey player is weighed down by their gear, hockey pucks do not have enough momentum, and hockey players brace hard against the ice, exerting too much force on the ice for a puck to take them backwards. The author hypothesizes that sending a puck at Mach 8 still would not work as it would likely melt, lose half its momentum before reaching the player, and/or explode upon impact.

# Question 27: If everyone on the planet stayed away from each other for a couple of weeks, wouldn't the common cold be wiped out?

First of all, stopping all types of economic activity for a few weeks would cost trillions of dollars in output, causing a global economic collapse. Also, it would be difficult to get people far enough away from each other as we would only be able to separate—at most—77 meters from each other and even then we would need to place people in uninhabitable areas of the world.

In answering if it would actually cure the cold, the author explains that after a week or two, the rhinovirus that causes colds would be eliminated from our bodies and die out: in a healthy immune system. However, those that have severely weakened immune systems will likely hold on to these rhinoviruses for weeks, or even months, and the common cold would be back as soon as these people rejoined the human population.

# Question 28: What if a glass of water was, all of a sudden, literally half empty?

Munroe first defines that a half empty glass is actually filled with water and air. So, to explain, he demonstrates three glasses: one with air/water, one with water/vacuum (absence of anything), and one with air/water, but with the bottom half holding air. In this scenario, the water/vacuum glass (the one demonstrating his answer to the question) would begin to boil and fill with water vapor, which will eventually fill with air and cause a slight shockwave as the vacuum collapses. Essentially, this would destroy the glass, and the other two next to it.

## Question 29: Let's assume there's life on the nearest habitable exoplanet and that they have technology comparable to ours. If they looked at our star right now, what would they see?

Ultimately, they would see nothing. The author explains that they may be able to pick up some of our radio transmissions. This would not be TV and radio like we traditionally believe, but rather early-warning radar left over from the Cold War. The visible light from our planet, from the Sun's light reflecting off our surface and back into space, could possibly be detected, but it would really only tell them what our atmosphere is like and not much else.

# Question 30: This may be a bit gruesome, but…if someone's DNA suddenly vanished, how long would that person last?

A person would be a third of a pound lighter. Then, he explains the medical effects via explaining what a *Amanita bisporigera* mushroom, or destroying angel mushroom, does upon ingestion. Your body experiences cholera-like symptoms, which mysteriously go away as you begin to feel better. While this is happening, the amatoxins that the mushroom are being released and are binding to the enzymes that read your DNA, interrupting their processes. This causes—among other things—liver and kidney failure.

The author also compares the effects of losing your DNA as similar to receiving radiation and chemotherapy treatments, which cause cell death and the collapse of the immune system. It is likely that losing your DNA would cause you to experience horrible physical symptoms until you die within a few days or hours.

# Question 31: What would happen if you tried to fly a normal Earth airplane above different solar system bodies?

First, we would need to use an electric motor for our plane as gas engines need oxygen in the air to run, and not every planet has oxygen in it's atmosphere. Examining the effects on 32 of the largest bodies in our solar system, most have no atmosphere so the plane would fall straight into the ground. Only nine have a thick enough atmosphere.

On the Sun, the plane would be vaporized. On Mars, it would not be able to move fast enough to stay in the air and the crash would be fatal. On Venus, the plane would fly, but it would be on fire and fall apart pretty quickly. On Jupiter, the plane would continue to sink down through the gas and liquid levels until it was crushed. On Saturn, the plane would maintain flight for a little while, but it's ending would be similar to that on Jupiter. On Uranus, you have the best chance of flying for a while, but it would be boring as the surface is featureless. On Neptune, the plane would freeze or break apart from ice turbulence. And on Titan, the airplane would actually fly easier than on Earth, but it would be so cold on this planet that you would need a plane specially fitted for it's temperatures.

# Question 32:_How much Force power can Yoda output?

To answer this question, the author draws on the scene where Yoda lifts Luke's X-wing from the swamp. Using a few guesstimates (as well as rabid fans' obsessive cataloguing of the surface gravity of each planet in *Star Wars*), he calculates Yoda's peak power output as 19.2kW, or enough Force power to provide electricity for a block of suburban homes.

# Question 33: Which U.S. state is actually flown over the most?

The author examined over ten thousand air traffic routes to respond to this question and finds that the most passed over state is Virginia. The largest factor behind this is the Hartsfield-Jackson Atlanta International Airport, which is the busiest in the world and is responsible for 20 percent of all flights that cross Virginia. The Toronto Pearson International Airport is also responsible for this statistic as they have the most direct flights to the Caribbean and South America, which has airspace right over Virginia.

The state with the highest ratio of flight-over-to-flight-to is Delaware, mostly because it does not have an airport. The least flown over state is Hawaii (or California, if you are sticking to non-island states).

**QUESTION 34: WHAT IF I JUMPED OUT OF AN AIRPLANE WITH A COUPLE OF TANKS OF HELIUM AND ONE HUGE, UN-INFLATED BALLOON? THEN, WHILE FALLING, I RELEASE THE HELIUM AND FILL THE BALLOON. HOW LONG OF A FALL WOULD I NEED IN ORDER FOR THE BALLOON TO SLOW ME ENOUGH THAT I COULD LAND SAFELY?**

Technically, if the balloon were 10-20 meters across and filled with air (not helium) you could use it as a parachute. If using helium, you would need at least ten 250 cubic feet helium tanks to fill a balloon to support your weight, and you would need to fill it fast for it to work.

# Question 35: Is there enough energy to move the entire current human population off-planet?

There is enough energy in the world, but it is not possible to apply it all. The author examines several ways of getting the Earth's population off-planet: such as rockets, a "space elevator," or even some sort of nuclear pulse propulsion, but ultimately we would use up all of our resources and possibly destroy the planet in our attempts.

## Question 36: I read about some researchers who were trying to produce sperm from bone marrow stem cells. If a woman were to have sperm cells made from her own stem cells and impregnate herself, what would be her relationship to her daughter?

If a woman had a child with herself, it would essentially be inbreeding and cause something called homozygosity. This could lead to many genetic disorders such as spinal muscular atrophy and sickle-cell anemia. Even further, the child would essentially be a clone of their parent, but be missing half of their chromosomes, causing severe genetic damage.

# Question 37: How high can a human throw something?

Humans have the greatest accuracy and precision of throwing something than all the rest of the animal kingdom, but we throw things better forward than upward. The world record is held by Roald Bradstock, a British javelin thrower who was able to throw a golf ball 170 yards.

# Question 38: How close would you have to be to a supernova to get a lethal dose of neutrino radiation?

The author points how strange this question is, as it is mixing neutrinos and supernovae, which are on two completely different scales. Neutrinos barely even interact with matter at all, so it would be difficult to have one affect a human, let alone enough to hurt someone. Supernovae, on the other hand, are unimaginably large. However, during a supernovae, the collapse of a stellar core into a neutron star actually releases neutrinos, but not nearly enough to cause any injury from radiation.

# Question 39: How fast can you hit a speed bump while driving and live?

No matter how fast you hit a speed bump, the jolt itself will not injure you as your car's suspension protects you against that. If the bump hits the frame of the car, the wheel rims, or any other part than the tires, then it is likely that your car will be extremely damaged (think: exploding tires).

To fully examine this scenario, the author imagines a car that is somehow able to go faster than its top speed (air resistance being the deciding factor). If a typical sedan were to go between 150-300 mph, the air resistance would literally lift it off the ground, cause it to tumble, and crash—all before the car even reaches the bump.

## Question 40: If two immortal people were placed on opposite sides of an uninhabited Earthlike planet, how long would it take them to find each other? 100,000 years? 1,000,000 years? 100,000,000,000 years?

If you assume that they would need to be within a kilometer of each other, and that they are walking around at random for a full twelve hours a day, the author calculates that it would take 3,000 years. This, of course, does not take in to account the visibility of the environment—so they may actually need to be closer. The author also postulates whether the people are actually searching at random or have some sort of strategy. To answer this, he provides several different ways in which these two people could hypothetically meet, and they ultimately result in the meeting taking place anywhere between five years to decades.

# Questions 41-43: Orbital speed

What if a spacecraft slowed down on reentry to just a few miles per hour using rocket boosters like the Mars sky crane? Would it negate the need for a heat shield?

Is it possible for a spacecraft to control its reentry in such a way that it avoids the atmospheric compression and thus would not require the expensive (and relatively fragile) heat shield on the outside?

Could a (small) rocket (with payload) be lifted to a high point in the atmosphere where it would only need a small rocket to get to escape velocity?

The author answers all three of these questions together because they all hinge on one main issue: getting into orbit is about speed, not height. Because gravity even near Earth's orbit is just as powerful as gravity on the surface, you really only can avoid it by going very fast in a sideways direction. The exact speed is about eight kilometers per second which is much faster than even a bullet travels. The biggest problem in reaching orbit is that it takes much more fuel to reach the speed requirements, not the height.

# Question 44: When—if ever—will the bandwidth of the Internet surpass that of FedEx?

Munroe estimates that currently FedEx is capable of transferring a hundred times the current output of the Internet. Using Cisco estimates, he explains that as the Internet is growing at about 29% a year, it will reach FedEx numbers by 2040; but, by then we will have much better data storage sizes, so that probably will not happen. Ultimately, the Internet is unlikely to beat FedEx's numbers.

# Question 45: What place on Earth would allow you to free-fall the longest by jumping off it? What about using a squirrel suit?

The largest vertical drop on Earth is on Canada's Mount Thor, where it would take about 26 full seconds to fall from top to bottom. Using a wingsuit, a person will fall much slower, losing altitude at around 18 meters per second (rather than 55 if freefalling). This would extend a person's fall to a minute. The record for longest wingsuit BASE jump is three minutes and twenty seconds, from Mount Eiger in Switzerland.

# Question 46: In the movie *300* they shoot arrows up into the sky and they seemingly blot out the sun. Is this possible, and how many arrows would it take?

He actually considers four different ways in trying to make this work. First, he considers longbow archers who can fire eight to ten arrows per minute. Even packing them into twenty rows, with two archers per meter, there will still only be eighteen arrows in the air at one moment: not nearly enough to block the sun.

In the second scenario, he packs the archers much more tightly and uses 130 archers per meter firing at seven arrows for every eight seconds. With this, still only 1.56 percent of the sun would be blocked.

The third attempt considers using Gatling bows, which fire arrows automatically and can fire 70 arrows per second. He ups this to forcing 300 arrows per second and calculates that it would block out 99 percent of the sun.

Munroe's easiest solution is the final one where he considers not that the Sun is in midday sky, but rather at the eastern horizon. This way, if the archers were firing north, then the shadow effect could accomplish this easily.

# Question 47: How quickly would the oceans drain if a circular portal 10 meters in radius leading into space were created at the bottom of Challenger Deep, the deepest spot in the ocean? How would the Earth change as the water was being drained?

Munroe calculates that it would take hundreds of thousands of years for the ocean to drain. This is because even though the opening is huge, the oceans are much larger. He suggests opening more drains to allow the water to drain faster and then examines each drop in meters and how it would change the world map. It is not until a loss of 200 meters that the map begins to truly change: with small islands appearing and the Netherlands dominating Europe. At a loss of one kilometer of water, the Arctic Ocean is cut off from the drain, the waters stop being depleted, and North America will be connected to

Europe. By five kilometers loss, most of the major oceans are disconnected from the drains and will lose no more water. In this scenario, our atmosphere and environment would suffer greatly and likely cause mass extinctions.

# Question 48: Supposing you did drain the oceans, and dumped the water on top of the *Curiosity* rover, how would Mars change as the water accumulated?

Even though water on Mars is frozen, we would be dumping so much warmer water so fast that it would turn Gale Crater (where *Curiosity* currently sits) into a lake. This would continue to flow until Mount Sharp (a peak in the middle of Gale Crater) would become an island, and then be covered completely. Water would continue to pool out into the North Polar Basin, and eventually fill even the Valles Marineris. Once we have finally emptied the water that would have left Earth (remember, there would still be water left on Earth from our previous question), only a few volcanoes, such as Olympus Mons, would remain above sea level. Eventually, these oceans would freeze and migrate to the permafrost at the poles.

# Question 49: How many unique English tweets are possible? How long would it take for the population of the world to read them all out loud?

The biggest issue to consider here is that the Tweets need to be understandable English words (ignoring that incomprehensible words might be proper nouns, such as names). The author explains the idea that information is tied to how uncertain a recipient might be to a message and their ability to predict it. He provides a mathematical equation based on this idea and comes up with the number two times ten to the forty-sixth power.

To read them all out loud, it would take a person ten to the forty-seventh power seconds, or ten thousand eternal years—much longer than the lifetime of Earth.

# Question 50: How many Lego bricks would it take to build a bridge capable of carrying traffic from London to New York? Have that many Lego bricks been manufactured?

To simply connect the two cities, you would only need 350 million of them and there have been over 400 billion Lego blocks produced. However, to build a bridge that could support traffic, it would need to be wider and deeper (and likely be made of the 2x4 bricks) and be covered in a sealant to make them denser in the water. Making this bridge is not possible as there are not nearly enough Lego pieces in existence. Also, this bridge would be subjected to extreme weather from the North Atlantic, so there may need to be some sort of anchor to help keep the bridge from drifting off. More anchors and weights would need to be added to avoid it sinking from waves and ultimately, it would need to reach the sea floor. This would stop the flow of the North Atlantic Ocean.

Even the easiest bridge plan (the simple connecting idea) would cost over $5 trillion.

# Question 51: What is the longest possible sunset you can experience while driving, assuming we are obeying the speed limit and driving on paved roads?

First, the author provides the definition that a sunset begins the moment the Sun touches the horizon and ends when it has completely disappeared. He also pays very close attention to the question's specification of a paved road, eliminating areas likes the South Pole. So the closest road to either pole (because they experience the longest sunsets) is in Longyearbyen in Norway. The longest sunset you can experience here is just short of an hour. Munroe's suggestion is to wait for a day when the day-night line is in your position in Norway and once it reaches you, drive north to stay a little bit ahead of it, then make a U-turn and drive back south quickly. This will result in a sunset as long as 95 minutes.

## Question 52: If you call a random phone number and say "God bless you," what are the chances that the person who answers just sneezed?

It is likely about one to 40,000 and he roughly arrives at this number through data from a doctor interviewed on ABC News. The doctor in his interview estimated that the average person sneezes around 200 times per year. Munroe does not recommend you conduct this experiment, however, as you are much more likely to be blessing a person who just murdered someone than a person who just sneezed.

# Question 53: How long would it take for people to notice their weight gain if the mean radius of the world expanded by 1cm every second?

As the Earth begins to expand you would feel a small, brief jolt. After the first day, the Earth will have expanded by 864 meters, and after a month it will have expanded by 26 kilometers, increasing it's mass by 1.2%. You would not really notice any change in weight, but you would begin to physically see the expansion of the Earth through cracks in the foundation. After a year, gravity would be 5% stronger and you would begin to notice not just weight gain, but the failure of roads, bridges, power lines, and satellites. The air would begin to be heavier as our atmosphere would not be expanding with the surface.

After five years, gravity is 25% stronger and you could weigh up to 18kg more. After ten years gravity is up 50% and the air in our atmosphere would be so thin we would have difficulty breathing. After 40 years we would have difficulty walking. And after 100 years we would be completely unable to move and our hearts would be unable to pump blood due to the immense gravity of the Earth. At some point, the Earth would collapse into a white dwarf or neutron star.

## Question 54: Assuming a zero-gravity environment with an atmosphere identical to Earth's, how long would it take the friction of air to stop an arrow fired from a bow? Would it eventually come to a standstill and hover in midair?

After flying very far, the air resistance would slow down the arrow and stop it. It would stay in the air, but after a few hours it would be moving so slowly that you could not tell it was moving at all. By this point, it would have traveled much farther than an arrow in regular gravity—at least five to ten kilometers.

# Question 55: What would happen to the Earth if the Sun suddenly switched off?

The author points out that this is the single-most asked question he receives, so he has a very detailed explanation for his answer, which highlights all the positives results of this.

He begins with solar flares and discusses how there would be a reduced risk of them. We would also experience improved satellite service as our communications satellites would no longer pass in front of the Sun. With less atmospheric noise, astronomers would be able to observe the stars around the clock. Because the Sun is gone, our water would turn to ice and we would no longer need bridges, therefore saving billions of dollars on infrastructure repairs. Due to no more time zones, business would run much smoother and thus be less expensive. With no direct sunlight, babies would be safer. Sneezing due to the Sun would be eliminated and potentially save combat pilots during flight. And finally, a chemical released by parsnips (which is activated by sunlight) would no longer be dangerous.

All of these benefits, of course, are pointless as without the Sun we would all freeze and die.

## Question 56: If you had a printed version of the whole of (say, the English) Wikipedia, how many printers would you need in order to keep up with the changes made to the live version?

Essentially, it would take only six printers. To print the entire encyclopedia of Wikipedia, it is estimated that the volumes would fill several bookshelves. The hardest part would be to keep up with the edits. The English Wikipedia receives around 125 thousand to 150 thousand edits every day. To keep up, these six printers would be running constantly, printing 15 pages a minute, and between the electricity, paper, people managing the printers, and the ink, it would cost a half a million dollars every month.

## QUESTION 57: WHEN, IF EVER, WILL FACEBOOK CONTAIN MORE PROFILES OF DEAD PEOPLE THAN LIVING ONES?

Most Facebook users tend to be young but based on the age breakdown of it's users over time, it is estimated that there are about 10-20 million people who have created profiles who are now deceased. The date where the dead will outnumber the living is entirely dependent upon the popularity of Facebook in the future. If Facebook begins to decline in users later this decade, the crossover date will be around 2065. Yet, if it remains continuously a part of social media as it is today, then the crossover date could be near 2100.

# Question 58: When (if ever) did the Sun finally set on the British Empire?

Technically, it has not and will not. This is because Britain has 14 overseas territories that are remnants of the British Empire. The Sun can physically never set on all 14 of these territories at once. There is one tiny set of islands, the Pitcairn Islands in the South Pacific, that are the holdout and if the UK ever loses them, then the Sun truly will set after over two centuries. The only chance of this happening otherwise is if a total eclipse passes over the islands at the right time of day, but this could take millennia.

**QUESTION 59: I WAS ABSENTMINDEDLY STIRRING A CUP OF HOT TEA, WHEN I GOT TO THINKING, "AREN'T I ACTUALLY ADDING KINETIC ENERGY INTO THIS CUP?" I KNOW THAT STIRRING DOES HELP TO COOL DOWN THE TEA, BUT WHAT IF I WERE TO STIR IT FASTER? WOULD I BE ABLE TO BOIL A CUP OF WATER BY STIRRING?**

Even though the basic idea makes sense, the answer is no. This is because it takes a huge amount of energy to heat water, upwards of 700 watts to heat a cup of water in two minutes. This is the same amount of energy output as a microwave, so really, the author suggests you are better off using the microwave.

## Question 60: If all the lightning strikes happening in the world on any given day all happened in the same place at once, what would happen to that place?

If this happened and all the lighting bolts came down in parallel together as one large channeled bolt, it would be comparable to two atomic bombs. Light and heat from the bolt would ignite the environment for miles and the resulting shockwave would flatten everything on nearby surfaces.

The author explains that there is one place on Earth, in Venezuela, where thunderstorms form nearly every night and generate lightning around every two seconds. If this were able to be harnessed, it would store up enough electric energy to power a gaming console and television for a hundred years.

# Question 61: What is the farthest one human being has ever been from every other living person? Were they lonely?

According to the author, the most likely answer is when the six Apollo command module pilots were in lunar orbit during the Moon landing. Each one stayed alone in the module while the other two were on the Moon, making it about 3585 kilometers from another human being. The Polynesians were likely to have come close to this as they spread across the Pacific and perhaps a sailor accidentally rushed ahead, but it is not possible to know for sure. The author also suggests Robert Falcon Scott, a British explorer of Antarctica whose expedition to the South Pole ended in the death of all but one crewman. But, that man was still within 3585 kilometers of another person.

To answer if they were lonely, Munroe shares an experience from one of the Apollo astronauts' book. In it, he basically states that he was alone, but not lonely. Rather, he felt he was a part of a larger experience.

# Question 62: What if a rainstorm dropped all of its water in a single giant drop?

If the storm measured 100 kilometers, then the water in that storm would weigh 600 million tons. A drop this heavy would fall at 90 meters per second. This massive drop would obliterate everything beneath, and around it, for at least a few kilometers. The splash from this drop would demolish everything within 20-30 kilometers and there would be flash flooding in those surrounding areas for nearly hours afterwards. Munroe nicknames this the dubstep storm due to the effect when the drop hits.

# Question 63: What if everyone who took the SAT guessed on every multiple choice question? How many perfect scores would there be?

Because each multiple choice question has five options, a random guess has a 20% chance of being correct. So, to get all 158 questions right, there is a probability of one in 27 quinquatrigintillion: which basically means it is impossible.

# Question 64: If a bullet with the density of a neutron star were fired from a handgun (ignoring the how) at the Earth's surface, would the Earth be destroyed?

This bullet would weigh as much as the Empire State Building, fall straight through the ground, and immediately pass through the crust of the Earth. This is because neutron stars are one of the most dense objects in existence. If the bullet were to pass through the Earth, the author suggests, it would be the first underground shooting star. But, it would likely stop once it reached the nickel-iron core of the Earth. If you attempted to touch the bullet, the force of gravity would be so strong that your blood would literally break through your skin and pour out of your fingertips, creating a blood sphere around the bullet.

## Question 65: What if a Richter magnitude 15 earthquake were to hit America at, let's say, New York City? What about a Richter 20? 25?

A magnitude 15 earthquake would release ten to the thirty-second power joules of energy, which is nearly the same amount of power as Earth's gravitational pull. The author does not answer this question any further, but rather demonstrates situations that are the equivalent of earthquakes on the opposite end of the scale: from zero and below, ending the book on an unusually upbeat response.

# ANALYSIS

This work offers a humorous and educational look at some of the strangest questions humans have had about the world around them. A lot of what the author provides through his answers is scientific, but through his clever voice and amusing stick-figure cartoons, his responses are easily accessible to even the most non-scientific mind.

A strength of the book is the humor. Munroe, while obviously extremely intelligent as he worked at NASA, does not claim to be an expert in any of these areas. Yet, he draws from other experts (such as people working in the math and science fields, journals, press releases, etc.) to respond to these questions. In doing so, it would be extremely easy to provide answers that are full of dry scientific information, and not much else. Munroe does not do this, however, and draws on his own colorful personality, and skills as a web comic cartoonist, to provide hilarious and educational answers. A reader of this book can easily come out of this with a newfound knowledge of several math and physics related topics without ever feeling like they were being forced the information.

One of the foundational assumptions of this book is that the reader will share an interest in understanding the concepts that these questions cover. One of the best aspects of this book is that readers do not need much previous knowledge in the scientific field, but it is assumed that if one is reading this book, that they too are curious about some of these hypothetical questions.

Criticism of this book might come from people who think that Munroe does not take some of these scientific principals seriously enough. After all, some of his responses are entirely through cartoons. In some cases, his footnotes or [citation needed] remarks (which are meant to add to the humor in his response) might bother certain overly analytical minds who genuinely want the sources or data further explained. Ultimately, this book is meant to be a humorous collection of absurd questions and answers, so people expecting a completely serious response to these topics should look elsewhere.

Having said that, the quality of research in this book is top notch. Having been a former scientist, Munroe understands the importance of backing up his answers, and provides a twenty-three page reference section detailing each source used in his individual responses. Not only does this add to the author's credibility as he provides the data that backs up his responses, but it also allows the reader to follow these sources for themselves if they care to examine a particular topic further.

What the reader can take from this book is an easily understood and humorous education on certain mathematical and scientific related topics. After having read this, the audience can go on to explain strange and interesting things such as why certain elements in the Periodic Table would be too volatile to place next to each other, or precisely how much Force energy Yoda from *Star Wars* can truly generate. The benefit to everyday life is pretty minimal, but it does provide the reader with a plethora of interesting factoids to share with family and friends.